SIMEN BLISS

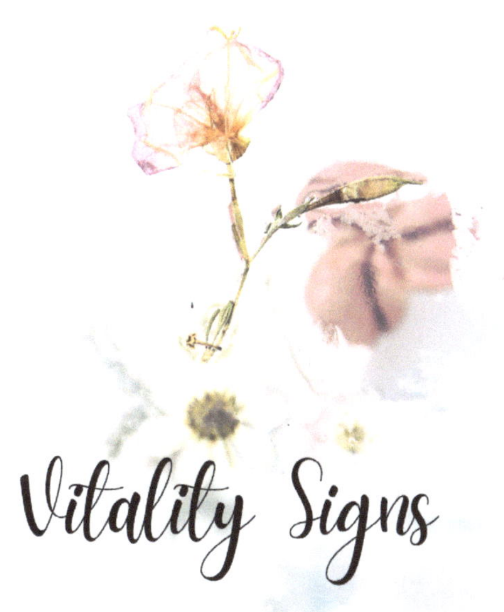

Vitality Signs

How to Increase Vitality Signs: Fullness,
Hair Growth, Eyelashes, Skin etc.

Vitality Signs

How to Increase Vitality Signs: Nutrition Stores, Hair Growth, Eyelashes, Skin etc.

Vitality Signs: How to Increase Vitality Signs:
Nutrition Stores, Hair Growth, Eyelashes, Skin etc.
Simen Bliss
Edition 1.1
Published 1. June 2022

Disclaimer

All this info is for entertainment purposes and based upon my personal experiences and beliefs. You are always responsible for your own wellness and vitality. These are my viewpoints and opinions as I feel it is with all information after having focused on ideal nutrition for 12 years.

This book is sold for information purposes only. Neither the author, the publisher, nor the distributors will be held accountable for the use or misuse of the information contained in this book. This book is not intended as medical advice because the author and publisher of this work do not recommend the use of cooked foods or medicines to alleviate health challenges. Because there is always some risk involved, the author, publisher and/or distributors of this book are not responsible for any not positive effects or consequences resulting from the use of any suggestions or procedures described in this book.

Intro

The body is created primarily with the foods we eat, what we breathe, drink and absorb through the skin.

So, the body is primarily created with what we eat.

Natural foods and processed foods store completely differently in the body. Beneficial foods only increase nutrition stores such as breasts, buttocks, hair, skin and muscles, while processed foods store as what people call fat.
It is natural to have a yin layer for women, while men have more visible abs, but by eating foods that are natural, it stores in beautiful ways. At the same time, we should not push fats, such as eating whole nut butters, but rather increase fruit amounts. Some fat is good, but dont push fats.
Because, the first realization is that most people can get more nutrition, but in clean forms, but be gentle with the fats, as in not eating whole nut butter jars just for getting more nutrients, although some is good, because this is better for the body, so just eat some fats in normal amounts and this is good, but eat more fruits and greens for example, as well as a wide variety with foods and learn the principles in this book, and then go with your intuition. In this book you learn how much you can actually affect your vitality signs.

It is about eating a lot, eating clean, and also eating in ways that are easy to absorb, while eating the right things, and learning what is truly nourishing for you, and including more variety and learning that some herbs are especially beneficial for certain things. It is about all the things summarizing to the total results.

For example, eyelash length is similar to flower length or leaf length.

The more elements we gather in clean form, the more our eyelashes grow, the more voluminous hair on the head we have and the more vitality signs we have, like breast fullness, buttocks size, relatively tone stomach, sparkly eyes, glowing skin, smooth skin, hydrated plump skin, muscle growth, skin color around the eyes and elastic youthful skin. These signs show our nutritional status, although genetics does influence as well.

A big reason why vitality signs make sense to learn how to enhance, is that they are exactly that, vitality signs. By having learnt this information, you have learnt more about how to enhance your vitality.

Enhancing is actually about giving the body what is right for the body, so it is actually about being in ideal balance, and ideal balance is ideal vitality.

A different word for nutrition is prana. It is really about being full with prana, but through balanced nutrition.

Imagine if millions or billions read this book, and so many more people become much more vital.
Imagine how this affects society.
The effects are really much greater than what most people think if we enhance people's nutrition. Food influences behavior, and food affects how positive impacts we have on the world.

You may already be vital, but there are greater and greater stages according to how greatly we implement nutrition, and by choosing to read this book, you are very likely to be vital or super vital in this life according to how inspired you are, but always feel your intuition for what is the absolutely best for you.

Set point

When you focus on vitality signs, the vitality signs you focus on are actualised more because you automatically do things that make them happen more and you have attracted and attract more things that benefit what you focus on.

Foundations

The foundations are essential for all vitality signs.

The foundations include plenty fruits and greens, plus other amino containing foods and variety.

To make it more interesting, I will write the other foundations within the vitality signs where they are most essential, and summarize them after.

Nutrition

The body places nutrition in many places and uses energy and some minerals according to requirements.

Extra elements become more bone density, more elements inside the bone marrow, more plump skin, more hair on the head, more eyelashes and so on.

Hydrogen is an element, iron is an element, silica is an element etc.

Women places more nutrients in the breasts and buttocks as breast milk and beneficial mass, while men have extra prioritization for height and muscles.

Women can be very muscular and athletic anyway, and women can also be tall, but the general difference is that women place more additional mass in the breasts and buttocks in addition to muscles, and certainly there are more things affected by biological gender. The clean mass in the breast and buttocks is not the same as what could be created with artificial candy, it is clean elements and energy.

So, when eating well, the extra nutrition goes into the breasts, buttocks, hair or becomes extra energy, also in accordance with what the body is prioritizing.

The body prioritizes different things according to hormones, and both men and women require both testosterone, progesterone and estrogen, but in different ratios.

Absorption

Most people absorb well, but some people benefit by taking mastic gum every fifth day, supplement with zinc and centaury (centaurium erythraea) every day for a while so the stomach acid is strong.

Centaury can be mixed with stevia, and you can mix it in with other teas. Zinc is best with food. Mastic gum can be taken whenever during the day.

Breasts

It is super beneficial for a woman to have full breasts and it is a big reason as to why.

For complete actualization while in this Earth realm that we are living, being full with biophotons and elements is among the main things for full actualization, including our superpowers.

As the body is more full, more energy starts is added in and as the aura field in response to increased elemental mass and energy absorbed via clean foods, so having full breasts is just the start. The next stages are special.

The aura is also a vitality sign although you can affect the aura instantly through focus.

Breasts are similar to bank accounts. It is great to have full bank accounts with money.
Full breasts indicate that the body has all required elements to thrive, given the body is clean as well.

The breasts are the places for women where additional elements and energy are placed.

Breasts have elements (for example hydrogen, silica and all the elements that are beneficial) and energy.

Breasts also have energetically nourishing functions, so full breasts energetically makes people more generous and giving, given that they eat clean foods as well.

So, breasts are just showing how full women are with prana, and prana (sunlight biophotons plus other energies combined with elements) is what makes up the body.

It really is that simple.

You can always focus positively and this makes us feel better and benefits our lives as well, but being full with prana is what really makes you the most powerful, blissful and actualized real you.

However, it is only required to be consistent with nutritionally rich foods. Be moderate with nut butters for example, some fat is good, but when increasing amounts, rather indulge in completed and preferably original/wild fruits. Also, eat balanced and enjoy foods.
Just eat a gentle nutritional surplus, with many fruits and greens, and also some other foods

providing other nutrients, and be consistent. This is what causes full breasts, and balanced hormones.

The big thing here is that clean foods become beneficial mass for the body and actualizes us and junk foods would be placed in different places in the body and cleansed. Fruits add in beneficial ways and beneficial foods add in beneficial ways, in actualization your real you.

We are more than our body, and who we are in this life, but the food actualizes the body we have in this life.

The real you is you when you have all elements required for being you to the full, plus more factors. We are who we are anyway, including our bigger us, but we are much more actualized as we are more nourished in beneficial ways.

Herbs that increase prioritization for elemental energy in breasts include:

- Thai kudzu leaf (grown in a pot)

- Motherwort

- Blessed thistle

- Hops fermented in coconut water kefir or fermented fennel because it is so strongly alkaline.

- Fennel.

These herbs increase breast size in combination with a clean nutritional surplus as well.

These herbs are very yin, so feel for yourself how often you wish to eat them and use your intuition. They are often good to eat/drink in the evening every other day, as yin herbs are generally more relaxing. After you have used them for some months and consistently eat well, then eat these herbs sometimes, as you feel. Even though they increase prioritization for breasts, it also requires eating well and getting nutrients so you both can satisfy the requirement for moving, bones, hair, muscles, skin while also having more nutrition for breasts etc.

These herbs are very yin herbs, so if you for some reason feel like being more yang like running a race or something, then you can pause the herbs and you can also eat tribulus leaf or tribulus powder

Buttocks

In addition to the points mentioned about breast size, the buttocks also include much muscle although breasts also contain muscles.

The buttocks are the core muscles for athleticism in the body. Having muscles in the buttocks indicates that women and men are fit, and women also have additional mass in the buttocks.

Also, the shape indicates muscular balance and also genetics, and movements such as the "fire hydrant", "donkey kicks" and hip machine movements while arching and leaning forward, cause beneficial balance in the buttocks musculature, and this is beneficial for posture and athleticism. It is also very beneficial to do movements for the inner thigh muscles to balance the muscles in the buttocks and legs. The shape is affected by what movements are trained and how rich foods people are eating plus genetics.

It is great to have hip machines at home or make sure to use towels if using public gyms.

The reason that fire hydrant and hip machine movements are beneficial is that they make the movement patterns when doing other exercises such as squats more effective. The muscles use the strongest muscles in a movement pattern, so by making the side middle glute muscles strong, the glute is more active while doing squatting exercises etc, and it is better for athleticism and posture, and it is beneficial for the knees, and this is very beneficial for muscular balance. The reason quadruped leg raises are beneficial is because they cause better posture and it focuses on the glute muscles so they grow more than the quads, and this also benefits the squatting movements because the glutes are more engaged then, as the glutes are the strongest muscles in the body and beneficial to use while squatting.
Training the buttocks in multiple pathways also makes it more balanced.

Inner thigh leg lifts and standing up and touching the right foot with your left hand and then the left foot to your right hand is very balancing for the legs, especially when doing many middle glute movements.

Make sure to warm up and do gentle stretching.

When strength training, it is also very beneficial to train in many different ways to have a stable physique in multiple movement patterns.

How to enjoy training

By eating very well, training feels great. Also, train as much as feels comfortable until it is a habit. Adrenal enhancing herbs and core vitality herbs for energy make it a lot easier to train more.

These herbs, combined with eating well and sleeping well causes more energy:

Burdock

Burdock leaf grown in soil with azomite and iron is great for additional iron to the nutrition. It is also very beneficial for the circulatory system.

Dendrobium

Dendrobium must be combined with 3 liter coconut water and watermelon. The reason for this is that dendrobium is a super absorbent and pulls hydration into the body and you must be very full with coconut water and hydration at the same time to maintain the hydration in the skin when that happens, when it is absorbed.

Dendrobium causes more inner attraction, so the skin is more youthful looking. Dendrobium causes more inner hydration. The most essential is to drink 1 liter coconut water before and right after, and then drink the next liter within one hour, and then 1 liter the hour after that.

Coconut water is best to drink via glass or husk, but if drinking it via cartons, then mix in spirulina and b12 for certain reasons.
The inner hydration that dendrobium provides feels great, but always combine it with coconut water, and much coconut water, 3 liter.

This is a core youthfulness herb.

After some months where you have eaten dendrobium three times a month, I suggest only eating them once a month.

Astragalus, grown and eaten in legume pod form.

This herb increases "chi" or energy in the muscles and in the body, giving you more energy. Have it grown and eat it like a sugar snap pea, just as many as feels natural to pick. It is super worth it to have it grown. It is among the main longevity herbs as well.

Cleanliness

The cleaner our food is, the more vital we look.

Cleaner food cleanses and keeps the stomach area clean.

Clean foods are whole foods, while overly processed foods like bakery foods and artificial candy are unclean. Fortunately, there are many restaurants that provide super tasty meals and eating completed fruits taste even better. For example, it is possible to eat everything in a healthy version.

When eating many fruits and eating clean, the body cleanses, while prana stores in the breasts. This is how to have big breasts compared to stomach ratio. The most effective way to have big breasts while having a slim midsection is to eat well, train well, and eat mastogenic herbs. But also, realize that visible six packs are not necessary for most women, and anyway, it looks better to eat well so that the breasts and buttocks actually are full, by increasing the nutrition stores, and the only way to do that is to eat a lot. Women have a yin layer on the body, and men do too, but this then makes it so that men usually have more pronounced abs when in balance. Women still have toned stomachs when in balance, but the abs show more for men when in balance. There is a certain yin layer requirement that must be there before the breasts grow, so pushing for abs visibility for women is not suggested, but the stomach is toned and in shape.

When eating clean, the stomach is in shape, but it is not necessary to have a visible six pack for women, as mentioned, although it is good to train the core as well.

For men, visible abs indicates good hormonal levels.

The point is really just that by eating clean, you are in shape. A much better focus for women is to focus on enjoying as high quality foods as possible, including herbs and also focusing on training for having a strong buttocks and having nutrition stores in the breasts and buttocks. Some channels have promoted other things, but the truth is that the body focuses on fullness and this is beautiful. "BeYouToFull". Staying consistent with eating is the key to results. It is up to you to stay in truth even if propaganda channels show other things, and also to live your life in ways where you have the most positive influences. This is the main thing to comprehend, that natural foods store differently and the pattern that expands is different. More natural foods equals more breast size while the stomach is in shape, but not necessarily at the fitness competition levels where the women too often push too much the fat percentage to try to achieve some fake standard, while in reality the standard for females that are ideally vital is that the nutrition stores are full and the stomach is in shape, but not with very visible abs.

So, focus on growing breasts and buttocks in clean ways, and don't focus too much on having unnecessary low fat percentage as some industries try to promote, because females in balance have yin stores, but when eating clean, it stores in beautiful ways.

The breast compared to stomach ratio has to do with how much prana you absorb and how clean you are, not just genetics.

The only way to have really great skin is to be full with nutrition including hydrogen.

You can have both full breasts and a tone midsection.

The nutrition stores are a big aspect in what makes females look feminine.

To enjoy more cleanliness in foods, buy at the best sources you can, like fruit orchards, food forests, organic shops, whole foods shops etc, or have your own grown wild edible foods.

If you like a trim midsection, then focus on both training and cleanliness excellence, while eating well, this way you have both large breasts and a toned midsection. But realize, women, when in balance do have nutrition stores, and the cleaner you eat the more is stored in the breasts and buttocks.

So, is it possible to both have large breasts and a tone stomach at the same time?

Yes, but we must focus on training, cleanliness and nutritional fullness at the same time and accept the yin layer and nutrition stores. The yin layer is the beneficial thin layer for women on the stomach for example. It is not about a compromise, but accepting the thing yin layer to let the body be able to store more in the breasts, because the extreme fat percentages some women go to in some industries is not natural, but most essentially, it is about realizing that clean foods, truly nutritious foods, store completely differently and in much better ways. It is not even the same thing.

Hydrated plump skin

The skin stores elements like silica and hydrogen, and water containing fruits provide more hydrogen and beneficial elements to hydrate the skin.

Original coconut water is super beneficial for the skin, so drinking much original coconut water in husk or glass is the most essential thing.

The next most beneficial thing is mature original fruits because these are much fuller with beneficial elements and this benefits hydration.

Olives are great for the skin, but be gentle on the fat amounts, but include some fat sources.

Omega 3 containing sources are also beneficial.

The skin requires all elements, including aminos for collagen formation, hydration through fruit water and some beneficial fats.

Eating original mango is great for the skin as well because the high amounts with vitamin A benefit the skin and the full nutritional profile in mangoes is very rich and hydrating at the same time.

Much coconut water in glass or husk is also very beneficial.

Berries are also great for the skin.

Dried fruits and bread are best replaced with raw water containing foods. Some cooked foods may be alright, but the more raw foods you eat, the better, because raw foods have more water inside and contain enzymes. Enzymes cleanse the body, absorb and speed up processes.

Camu camu is also great for the skin, because it is super high in vitamin C, and vitamin C increases collagen production. Just half a teaspoon is great sometimes.

Aloe vera is very beneficial to in having hydrated skin too.

Eyes

Acai is great for making the eyes look fresh. The strong beautiful color makes the retinas more fresh.

Schizandra is also great for the eyes, and eucommia is great for the elasticity around the eyes. Schizandra positively affects an energy meridian visible in the eyes.

Dendrobium and hops and yin herbs are great for the skin color around the eyes. Dendrobium must be combined with 3 liter coconut water and something that causes blood vessel expansion like watermelon and beets.

Burdock is great for skin color around the eyes by providing more iron.

Eating many great iron containing foods habitually is essential for the areas around the eyes.

The areas around the eyes are best showing vitality by having internal attraction elements (dendrobium), iron fullness (burdock) and yin fullness (dendrobium).

Yin fullness is the skin plumpness that dendrobium mixed with much coconut water and watermelon benefits. We have a layer with hydration that also makes the face look youthful. These, plus many fruits, greens and also eating other foods in balanced amounts, makes great results happen and you may look surprisingly young.

This information is special.

You do this, and wow, the results are beyond great. It requires all the foundations.

The foundations are 3 big fruit meals and 3 other meals with more aminos, or somewhere around these amounts.

The fruit meals absorb easily, so they can be eaten an hour before an amino (protein) meal.

Being consistent with fruit and green amounts is the big key, as well as including more food types.

The skin color around the eyes is also benefited by having replaced wheat and yeast for something else.

The area around the eyes also requires good amounts with b12 so supplementing b12 sometimes is good.

Rose and hawthorne are also great for the eyes` shape.

Eyebright is also beneficial for eyes.

Be who you are

Be your essence. This has immense effects on your vitality as you get much more energy this way and it shows in a super positive way.

Be what you are in essence, and you feel this energetically.

Who you really are is perfection actualising itself as you, for what you are here for being. You also shape your experience through focus, so focus on the most positive things for you.

Eyes show our essence as well.

Be you and always listen to your intuition and instincts.

Hair

Hair on the head is among the biggest indicators for how rich nutrition we have absorbed, and are absorbing consistently, as well as hormonal balance.

It is especially beneficial to include certain herbs that boost hair growth and hormone balancing and nourishing herbs, but it absolutely requires eating nutritionally rich foods.

Hair is one way the body shows manna amount.

Organic foods are also much better for your hair because it benefits probiotics more and for other reasons, including hair color because organic foods contain more aromatic aminos that actually contribute to color in the hair.

The main thing is very much about realizing what actually provides you with elements, for example mature fruits instead of not mature fruits.

Hair herbs

Bhringraj:

Topically applying bhringraj on the head and washing it out while bending forward so it only touches the hair on the head, is beneficial for hair growth because it benefits the hair greatly both through cleansing, nourishing and prioritizing hair growth. Use it topically.

Polygonum multiflorum:

This herb is great for the hair and is best grown and eaten in leaf form, although it is often sold in root form. However, it is very similar to knotweed, and knotweed may not be allowed to grow in some regions in the United States, so check this before growing it outside, but if you can, it is a really beneficial plant for the hair, and it is really best in leaf form.

Mainly, hair growth is about having good amounts with nutrients in your body. So eating well consistently is the main factor.

Skullcap:

This herb benefits hair growth through a gentle increase in hair growth prioritization and hair nutrients.

Ecklonia cava:

This herb is very beneficial for hormonal quality and this benefits the hair. It is a seaweed, so it is best to eat it just every six days for keeping b12 absorption proper.

Saw palmetto:

This herb also is great for hormonal quality and this is very beneficial for the hair, especially in men.

Hormonal balance (usually having to include more yin herbs.)

Bamboo:

This herb is beneficial for the hair but the extract is very alkaline, so it is beneficial to have effective absorption and the centaury herb is beneficial for this. Whole bamboo shoots are usually absorbed well enough, but the extract is best to ferment for absorption reasons. Many shops including asian shops sell bamboo shoots.

Hops:

This herb is a very similar herb to bamboo in effect.

Because both provide so high levels with silica that they are so alkaline so it is beneficial to have effective absorption. This is different from greens where we can eat plenty of greens and this benefits the stomach acid, but from experience, bamboo and hops are best to ferment first.

Biotin can also be beneficial to add in for increased hair growth.

These steps benefit the eyelashes as well, but the eyelashes also benefit greatly with eating mineral rich foods and this is the main thing.

For men, learning how to preserve the prana is among the most beneficial things a man can do. Learning how to make the energy cycle in the body, and getting a satisfactory feeling in the head region instead, when being with a partner, is much more beneficial as all the nutrients then cycle into the body and add to the hair.

Polygala tenuifolia grown and eaten in leaf form inside or outside, is highly beneficial for men to cycle the energy in the sacral chakra up into the other chakras as it opens the energy channels between the sacral chakra and higher chakras more. The main thing for cycling the energy is how you focus the energy, focusing on the higher chakras, breathing, relaxing and spreading the energy in the body.

Yin herbs are beneficial for the hair, including motherwort and hops.

Eyelashes

Eyelashes are benefited by the same things as mentioned above in "Hair".

Mineral rich foods

Soaked nuts etc, provide much more bioavailable nutrients and minerals. So, if eating brazil nuts, make sure to put them in water first so the minerals become more biovailable.

Fruits that are mature (color has changed/aroma is present/texture is softer and taste is better) have more minerals and nutrients.

These two factors, have a big impact on how much minerals and elements you absorb.

Finding places that sell original/wild fruits is among the biggest things you can do for your vitality and youthfulness.

Smooth skin

For having smooth skin it is essential for some people to eat only tolerable foods, and replace nightshades, wheat, milk, eggs and onion (garlic might be a replacement for onion if used). This is essential for me for example so I have clean skin. It is also beneficial not to fry oils and replace refined sugar.

Milk thistle

A great herb to benefit you in having smooth skin is milk thistle because it cleanses the liver, so it is easier to keep yourself clean.

Schizandra

This is a great herb for the skin's beauty as well, it benefits the liver, kidneys and the whole body, as well as the skin. In Chinese herbalism, it is said that schizandra gives a present after having eaten it everyday for three months, and this is better skin. This herb contributes to having balance among all the energy meridians in the body.

Movement

Find a good PT so you have proper training form, and by eating well, including energizing herbs, training feels so great that you feel pleasure when training. It may require some momentum (training more times as well), but you do feel pleasure when you are nourished enough and have slept well, and have gotten into the rhythm.

Always warm up before training and include some posture exercises and do gentle stretching after working out.

Beneficial movements include warm ups, dancing, swimming, strength training, sprinting, going for walks, aerobic, jumping on trampolines, playing and much more etc.

Movement benefits the body in very many ways and is essential for vitality.

It makes the body absorb food better.

Movement cleanses your body.

Movement makes the skin look better.

Movement benefits mood.

Movement benefits circulation to the hair.

Train as much as feels comfortable, and increase weights etc, as feels great. Focusing on the training being enjoyable is what makes it a habit. As you have established a training habit, you can decide if you increase weights/repetions, but the main thing is to focus on enjoying it. Don't push reps, instead establish a love for training and do as many as feels great. The energy enhancing herbs makes you so energetic, when combined with the foundations, that it feels great.

Relaxation

Relaxation is great for all processes in the body. Both activity and relaxation, and also having fun and being relaxed while being active is great, although sometimes we may lift weights and that requires more energy, being relaxed during the day is very beneficial. We can be relaxed and highly active at the same time or just relaxed while sitting or laying.

Relaxation herbs include:

Mucuna (5 days on 1 day pause approximately), rose, hawthorn, holy basil, gotu kola, bacopa, schizandra and rhodiola rosea leaf or rhodiola sacra leaf (I like to use this one just sometimes because it is more serotonin focused and I like more ecstatic states, but it provides energy and relaxation for the future as well, so sometimes using it is great).

These herbs add real relaxation, and to be the most relaxed, it is very beneficial to be in places with beneficial frequencies.

Sleeping well and focusing on the most positive things, breathing, movement and gentle stretching and being our essence is very beneficial for our relaxation.

Being in our intuitive guidance and doing what we are inspired to is also central for relaxation.

Chamomile and lavender are also great to add, but the above mentioned ones plus lifestyle principles, make a bigger difference.

Sleep

Collagen production is approximately 30 times higher when sleeping.

Sleeping more shows in our fresh faces and is a clear vitality sign.

Earthing and swimming in the ocean

By touching the Earth with our skin, either ground, stone or ocean, we receive electrons that energize us and it relaxes us at the same time. We absorb some minerals while in the ocean, and our lymph system gets cleansed by the circulatory effects happening as well, in response to the shifting temperatures between comfortable ocean temperatures and the sun.

Patterns

We have multiple patterns that are actualised according to how great our nutrition is.

We have hydration patterns, iron patterns, mineral patterns for full hair growth, muscle growth patterns, nutrition store patterns and more.

The more they are actualised, the stronger the vitality sign. For example, luxuriant and voluminous hair is a strong vitality sign, muscle growth in the buttocks is a vitality sign, nutrition stores as the breasts and buttocks are vitality signs. These are patterns.

We also have patterns like the circulatory system which is more visible in men, with veins on arms showing that have good iron status, and this also affects skin color around the eyes. In essence, the body is multiple patterns stacked to form the body. Nutritional fullness is the cause for them all being actualised.

What to eat in a day

I like to keep this open regarding exactly what to eat to make it easy and to let intuition contribute.

For example, 3 fruit meals and 3 other meals containing more aminos is beneficial.

An essential thing about fruit meals, is that wild fruits that are completed (completely changed color etc), are much richer in minerals. In fact, green pineapples don't add minerals to the body but the body has to buffer the acids from the unfinished pineapples, so it is best, if eating green pineapples to combine them with greens in a smoothie. It is best to find completed fruits and necessary to achieve proper results. It is also better to eat wild original fruits, if you can find orchards that have wild original fruits because they provide much more minerals. When the fruits have more minerals, you get more minerals, and it is more hydrating because the acids are already buffered inside the fruit.

It may seem like some work to find a way to get all wild fruits, and you can have great vitality with hybrid fruits too, but wild fruits is really the higher level because you get so much more minerals per fruit. So, eventually, it is best to find a place that sells or has wild original edible fruits, but until then, it is certainly great to find fruits that are more completed, wherever you are.

I tell you the highest level, even if it may require more initially. You can also buy wild original fruit trees that are a couple years, or maybe you wish to move to a place that has more fruit trees.

This is something society must do better for all, and it is among the biggest guidelines in nature: to let the fruits be completed, and also to eat foods that originate in nature.

So, some people like to drink more smoothies and may mix greens with bananas or apples/pears, or have berry smoothies with acai and banana, or mango smoothies, or bananas with strawberry smoothies and so on. Eating a bowl with wild blueberries is also really great, and I love to eat bowls with wild blueberries. It is so positive and makes us look very fresh.

Raw foods are also better, but you can store up nutrition with some cooked meals as well. Raw foods are especially higher in levitational elements such as hydrogen.

A fruit meal may be a smoothie or a bowl with watermelon until you are satiated or papaya until you are satiated and so on. So, I eat as much fresh watermelon as I feel like when I eat it.

The fruits are very easy to absorb, so you can eat the fruit meal and then quickly eat another meal again after an hour, and this meal may contain more aminos or other nutrients.

It is very beneficial to eat a variety. Brazil nuts are for example super high in selenium, so including this sometimes is great. Most foods are very high in something, so by including a variety with foods according to your intuition, you are likely to get a great variety with foods in.

Iron often requires some focus for making sure you get in great amounts. If eating dates for iron, the best is to soak them first for a couple hours to preserve more moisture in the skin when eating them. I do suggest focusing on fruits that already contain the water inside, instead of putting dried fruits in water, because the fruits that already contain the hydrating fruit water inside are more hydrating than rehydrated fruits, but if you do eat dates sometimes, make sure to soak them before or eat them fresh. Strawberries, watermelon, chia seeds, legumes etc also contain iron, and many more foods.

Generally, red and black foods often contain more iron.
Camu camu is also very beneficial for absorbing iron.

The colors in food become vitamin A for use when required for example, and other nutrients and they maintain integrity in the skin and body and provide many benefits, and this is why this looks vital.

Glow up

When you eat plenty of color rich foods, the skin actually glows more.
Eating the rainbow is a super valuable and very foundational tip, and remains a super valuable tip combined with the special herbs mentioned in this book. How much color are you eating in a day?

Adding acai, adding strongly coloured fruits is so beneficial for the skin color.

Also, eating organic is better for the skin color because organic foods contain more aromatic aminos, and some among these aminos become the "tan" color we see. Some aminos become melanin.

Even though a tan is beneficial, be gentle with the skin when in the sun, because in the most nature there are many trees, making the light interspersed.

Certain edible foods like cactus flowers give a more sparkling effect in the skin as well, when combined with other factors. Flowers that sparkle add a sparkling effect to the skin, given the hydration and other food essentials are in place. Have you ever wondered why certain artificial makeups sometimes have sparkling effects? The sparkling effect that edible flowers have actually adds to your own sparkle in the skin.

To have great skin, it certainly is beneficial to be gentle about how much the face is in the sun, but it is natural to get some sun, so feeling the balance is beneficial.

So, regarding a color Glow Up, we see that by absorbing more aromatic aminos in organic foods, and color rich fruits adding more color, including implementing the foundations, and eating sparkly foods, we see this all adds to the total Glow in the skin. We also see that some edible flowers add a bright actual glow to our skin as well, especially in the sun, like bright edible flowers, and they do give glow, but it is best to cleanse them according to how clean the air is.

Visualisation

Visualize yourself as your most ideal version, nutritionally full and blissful and living your best life. This positively affects what you eat and attractions.

Affirmations

Say the affirmations you feel like saying, this positively influences your body to prioritize certain things and you in eating certain things.

Foundations summary

- Many fruits.
- Many greens that taste good.
- Including more food types for more nutrients and aminos.
- Water containing fruits, not dried fruits.
- Herbs. There are more I could mention, and for clients I suggest specific herbs for the clients for specific goals, but these are great general herbs for people, including herbs for specific things.
- Soaking nuts and seeds
- More raw foods.
- More fruits that are mature.
- Organic foods.
- Wild/original foods. The more foods that are original, among the foods you eat, the better.

Intuition

Always feel your intuition.

Also, focus on the positive and let your intuition guide you in living your best life.

www.ingramcontent.com/pod-product-compliance
Lightning Source LLC
Chambersburg PA
CBHW040929250726
48664CB00020BA/181